Changing Landscapes —*My New Normal*

A True Story of Struggle and Adjustment
after Surviving a Ruptured Aneurysm

Sarah Celio Krenk

ISBN: 978-1-4834-0506-3 (sc)
ISBN: 978-1-4834-0595-7 (hc)
ISBN: 978-1-4834-0544-5 (e)

Library of Congress Control Number: 2013920935

Lulu Publishing Services rev. date: 11/25/2013

Contents

Dedication vii

Introduction xi

Chapter 1: Growing Up 1

Chapter 2: Before 9

Chapter 3: The Event 19

Chapter 4: Inpatient Rehab 31

Chapter 5: Dark Days 37

Chapter 6: The Investigation Results 47

Chapter 7: Going Home 53

Chapter 8: Friends 59

Chapter 9: Invisible 65

Chapter 10: Tremors 69

Chapter 11: Tears and Travels 73

Chapter 12: Filters and Stressors 79

Chapter 13: Ugly and Dreams 83

Chapter 14: Coping 85

Chapter 15: Blessings 89

Chapter 16: Today 91

Dedication

I dedicate this book to my husband, Dan. I couldn't have endured this ordeal without your support (figuratively *and* literally) and encouragement. Thanks for putting up with my complaining and frustration. I know this situation is incredibly difficult for you, because you are dealing with it every day, just as I am.

Thank you Michelle, Stephanie, and Konni, for being unexpected shining stars in my life. I consider you all blessings. Your friendships make my struggles a little easier. I would like to thank Kevin (a.k.a. Kevil) for always being there to cheer me up when I am down in the dumps. I can always count on you to make me laugh. When Kimble got sick, when I got sick, when Dan was deployed, you were always a phone call away for help, and that is comforting. Thank you, Erica and Kevin, for countless rides to therapy.

I appreciate Suzanne for coming to my house and creating a "ghetto salon." Thank you, Kerri, Jill, Tacie, Steve B., Scott, and Lisa, for always standing as my pillars of support. I can always count on you for strength and cheerleading.

Thanks to my parents for your support, for your optimism, and for teaching me to have a strong spirit. Thanks to Amy at mycerebellarstrokerecovery.com. You have no idea how much you have helped me feel less alone. Unfortunately, you understand what I am going through first-hand, and you have become a friend whom I cherish. Your blog probably saved me from doing something drastic to myself! I would like to thank Chuck Orton for sending cards and asking what can be done to help. Your support from afar is very important to me. I would also like to thank my sweet friend, Aaron. Your love is like a beacon of light to me. I like how you don't treat me any differently now and you are so positive about my progress and accomplishments.

I want to thank Jennifer Perry, because I really feel like you are trying to understand. Your words and the words of the children you work with were so heartfelt, genuine, and encouraging to me. I love you all.

Thanks to my dad and Dan for helping me make this book a reality. It probably never would have been published without Dad's diligent hours of editing and Dan's help with the images. I want to thank my stepmother, Anne, for all of the faxes and helping me find a focus group. Thanks to Jean, Amy, Lisa S., Mary, and Heather F. for your time and input.

I could not have made progress without the support of Stacy Harwin. You are a beautiful person inside and out, and my life changed for the better the day I met you.

There is a little boy named Dalton, who is the son of one of the nurses where Dan is employed. Though I've never met him, he says a prayer for me every day. He has my picture in his room, and he lit a candle for me at his church this past weekend. I am grateful that he is thinking of me. I need all of the help I can get.

Introduction

This story isn't easy to recall, tell, write, or read. It has already been an incredibly long journey filled with joy and small victories and terrible frustration.

On March 11, 2012, I suffered one ruptured aneurysm, although I had two, and when the surgeons were "fixing" the aneurysms, with a surgical procedure called coiling, they induced a cerebellar stroke. Few people live through an event of this nature. The aneurysms almost killed me; the stroke caused long-term problems in the course of my recovery. This book came about because I have read a considerable amount of literature on the subject, and I realized that no two experiences are alike, yet there are some similarities with the struggles after a trauma. It helped me immensely to read about the experiences of others, and someone suggested that it is therapeutic to write.

I hope people read this experience and gain a better understanding of the struggles associated with a stroke. This story is far from over. I make small gains every day. I hope I do forever. This is a tale of hope and perseverance but also of great frustration.

I wrote this narrative to help anyone going through a life-changing illness; caretakers, friends, and family may gain greater insight into what it is like to struggle with recuperation. What you will get, if you choose to read this entire autobiography, is the truth of what I and many other people deal with day in and day out; what it is like to walk in my shoes. (I always joke that they are great shoes, but I can't wear heels now, so they are put away, for the time being. I was thrust into the world of Birkenstocks and flats with reliable traction. I bought a pair of low heels. I like to call them "training heels.")

What you won't get are lengthy definitions of strokes, aneurysms, or a lot of medical jargon. Chances are, anyone who has suffered through a similar medical trauma already knows technical definitions, but sometimes these victims don't want to dwell on the grim details. While reading and researching many books and blogs on these subjects, I have learned a few valuable lessons. The first is that no one's stroke or recovery is the same, so every piece of literature is unique. The second is that there is a common theme to the books and blogs: if their advice helps even one person understand or feel less alone, then their stories—and mine—are worth telling. When brain injury strikes, often the victim feels misunderstood, unsupported, and isolated. I hope my story helps someone.

Many books I have read take place many years into the recovery process. This chronicle started to form one year after my traumatic brain injury (TBI). The anger and frustration was fresh on my mind, but I think the beginning of recovery, and all of the negative feelings that accompany that time period, are important to document. It was a tumultuous period, but lately I think I have made great strides in a mere half a year.

I have no grand illusions of this being a bestseller, because this narrative doesn't necessarily apply to a wide audience. I originally only wanted to target my family and friends as readers, but then I realized this tale might be useful to a wider group of people. It just goes to show: life isn't all rainbows and fuzzy puppies. It is short and can change in the blink of an eye. This event has consumed my every second of every day for almost a year and a half, so forgive me if I sound negative at times. It is important that you, as the reader, get the truth, not a rosy version of the truth.

CHAPTER 1

Growing Up

I was born the day after Christmas in 1974. To me the best gift, to this day, is anything wrapped in birthday wrapping paper, not Christmas wrapping paper. My brothers could choose special birthday dinners that my mom would prepare. I had to eat pot roast, because my grandfather was always in town for the holidays, and he loved pot roast. I dislike pot roast to this day. My parents were expecting another boy. I was supposed to be Justin instead of Sarah. Surprise!

Before my injury, I had a good life. I grew up in Connecticut with my three older brothers, Matt, Steve, and Chris, and I had a pleasant childhood. The photograph that follows is my brothers and me in a happier time. My parents divorced when I was seven, but that didn't foster many unhappy memories. I spent pleasant times with my mom and grandparents on Cape Cod, eating seafood from beachside shacks (they always have the best food) and eating homemade coconut ice cream. My dad took us to many cities and many museums, and I learned about a wider world from him. We went camping on weekends in the summer and spent time at the beach, roughing it and absorbing the sunshine. I recall my dad reading aloud books by one of my favorite authors, Stephen King, and he did all of the voices of characters with their quaint and distinct accents. He would excel at reading books on tape. Scary stories probably weren't the best choice for a kid who was camping in the woods, but that's what I liked. The genres I most enjoyed were horror and comedies.

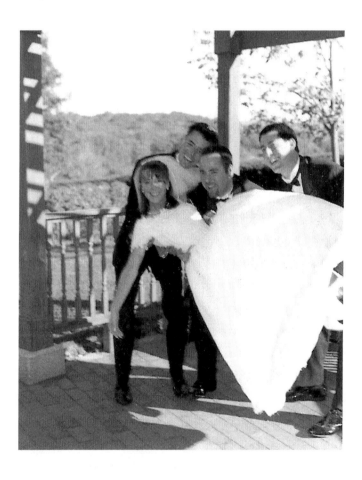

Pets were an integral part of our family. My first dog, Nikki, was a mean Shih Tzu. Someone came to our door and gave him to us. He mangled my brother's nose, but he was part of the family. Animals have affected my illness and recovery, which I will address later in my story.

My mother's mother, Shirley, was a doting grandmother. She loved having a granddaughter and liked to buy me girly clothes. Everyone wanted me in dresses and patent leather shoes because I was the only girl, but having three brothers, I was a tomboy. I preferred roughhousing or playing football to dollies, tea parties, or dancing. I started tap and jazz, reluctantly, when I was three, but I liked it so I kept on dancing until college. I even added hip-hop and lyrical ballet. It's hard to believe I did anything that required so much grace, because I was an accident prone and awkward child. In the sixth grade, I broke my arm in two places doing the limbo at a birthday party.

I didn't toss out all of my tomboy characteristics when I took up dancing; for instance, my fixation on football. My father, brothers, and I were fans of the St. Louis Rams team. I am still a big fan, and my brothers and I try to get to at least one game a year. When I got sick, Dan wrote and told the organization my story. I received an autographed helmet from the quarterback, Sam Bradford!

When my grandmother received her first Social Security check, she sent my brother, who was in college, one hundred dollars. She did that every month. After she passed away, my grandfather carried on that tradition with each of the four children. The day she died, my grandfather, great-grandmother, and I visited the family cemetery plot, and afterwards we ate hot dogs. Reflecting back, my grandmother frequently talked about death and she had reflected upon it that morning. I was nine years old. She had seen an all black butterfly and took that as a foreboding omen.

We were at my great-grandmother's house when my grandmother walked in from the porch and announced that she was dying. My grandfather had left to run some errands. The emergency line 911 wasn't established yet. I called Police Officer Looby, who often had spoken at my elementary school and had given us a phone number to call in case of emergency. I dialed that number from memory on the rotary phone in the kitchen. My grandmother had asthma, so I told them she was having an asthma attack. My great-grandmother was fanning her with a newspaper to get some air in. Her lips were turning a purplish-blue hue. A short while later, the police arrived and declared her dead on the scene.

I remember being eerily calm. I also remember her shrouded with a white sheet and seeing her hand twitch. I thought she was alive. Someone later said she died of a massive heart attack. I wonder now if it was an aneurysm and if there is a genetic proclivity in our family. I guess I will never know.

My grandfather, whom we called Bobby, was a laconic, stoic man. He worked for Colt, the gun manufacturer, and for Pratt & Whitney, creating airplane designs, primarily for World War II, then finished his forty-year career there. He was frugal and good at investing money. I loved spending the summers at his house on Cape Cod, going to the beach and the penny candy store. He had MTV, and we did not, so watching it was a big deal for my brother and me. We spent countless hours zoned out on music videos and reruns of *The Monkees*. We played croquet in his backyard quite a bit. My mom took good care of him as he aged. Bobby died in a nursing home after I graduated from college.

My grandmother on my father's side, Isabelle, was a piece of work. She was nervous, private, and ornery, but she was very funny and fiercely independent; I was probably closest to her. She would throw gifts in the garbage at Christmas right in front of us if she did not like or understand them. That was typical behavior we were accustomed to; we thought her antics were funny, not cruel. She would go to a restaurant and order a "burger with no nuts" (she had diverticulitis) or a "coffee with no hair." (I have no idea what that meant.) She would give me twenty dollars and say, "Go buy yourself a burger." She also sent a hundred dollars a month to each of the kids in college. I am realizing my grandparents kept me afloat! She loved her grandchildren and was a fun grandmother. Christmas Eve was a big occasion to her, and I remember her living room was always piled with gifts for everyone. It was tradition that we went there every Christmas Eve and ate pizza and then opened gifts. Back in the day, during the Cabbage Patch Kid craze, she told me she hit someone with her cane to win one for me. The thought of that made me laugh. She died after I graduated from college, also.

My grandfather on my father's side, Angelo, was a very cool man. He had silver hair. He played the saxophone in a jazz band and he taught me to play the clarinet, though I was never talented at that. I quit the school band some years later, and my dad went to a concert, expecting to hear me play. That was how he learned I had quit.

I recall singing with my grandfather. We always sang this: "Sarah, Sarah, sitting in a shoe shine shop. When she shines she sits all day. When she sits she shines all day. Sarah, Sarah, sitting in a shoe shine shop." Now sing it faster and faster. It's a tongue twister, and we laughed about it for hours. I remember when he was diagnosed with a brain tumor, and how he was in pain. He would hold his head and cry. That was so contrary to his typical jovial demeanor. He died when I was in the sixth grade.

My great-grandmother, Avis, was a big part of my childhood. She lived very close, and I spent most days after school at her house when my mother went to work. Every day she prepared an after-school snack for me of frozen pizzas or Ramen noodles, but she was a creative cook and baker too. I watched soap operas and sitcoms with her as she took her perch at her card table and played solitaire and smoked her Newport cigarettes. Wild animals were strangely comfortable in her presence. We used to feed birds, squirrels, and raccoons right out of our hands, like in a Disney movie. She died in a nursing home when I was a junior in high school. The photograph below is from the *Hartford Courant*, taken in a park by a passing newspaper photographer, when I was a child.

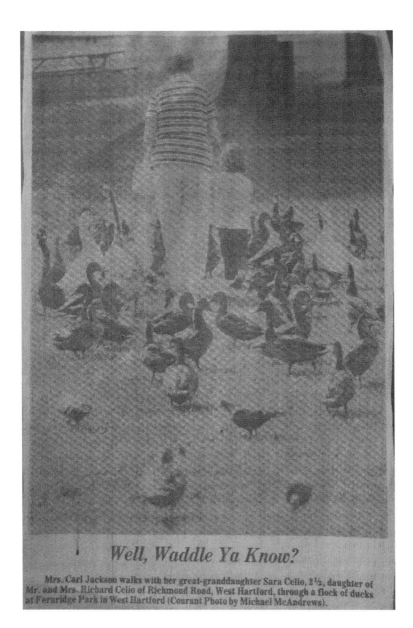

Well, Waddle Ya Know?

Mrs. Carl Jackson walks with her great-granddaughter Sara Celio, 2½, daughter of Mr. and Mrs. Richard Celio of Richmond Road, West Hartford, through a flock of ducks at Fernridge Park in West Hartford (Courant Photo by Michael McAndrews).

CHAPTER 2

Before

I went through an incredibly long awkward phase. Adolescence is hard enough, but I felt like an ugly duckling. My nieces and nephews never went through an awkward phase: they are all extremely good looking. I recall a picture my father took of me wearing a short, spiky haircut, in which I looked like the goat I was feeding in the photo. The nickname "Goat" stuck with me for years, snickered by my siblings, nieces, nephews, and even my high school boyfriend. My best friend growing up, Ami, was always gorgeous (though she might tell you differently). Ami moved away when I was in the third grade and she was in the fourth grade. We are still friends to this very day, which I think is a huge testament to our commitment to our friendship. There was no texting or e-mailing then, so it was rare for kids to stick together through distance and time.

High school was a blast. I went to a public high school. We have very good public schools in Connecticut. High school was more challenging for me academically than college or my graduate classes because I didn't apply myself academically: I was there for social time. My friends were very important to me, and I keep in touch with most of the people in our group now, although we were all different then and have chosen very different paths. I played field hockey and lacrosse, and I danced with the jazz dancers. There was a team of dancers in our high school who were intensely competitive. In order to be a part of that team, I had to audition every year. The photograph that follows is of my dance team (the girls in leotards were alternates).

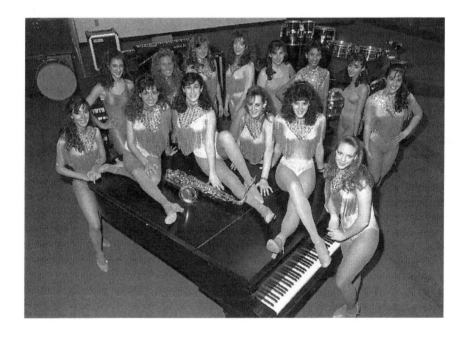

I contracted mononucleosis at the beginning of my senior year from drinking tainted water during field hockey practice, and I remember being so livid because I couldn't get to know a new boy who had come to our school. Everyone was intrigued with the new student. It is significant because some doctors have suggested that my aneurysms were triggered by a viral illness, perhaps a vestige of that mono infection. Other doctors disagreed. One day, the new boy said he was coming to visit me. In my juvenile mind, I thought I would impress him if I showed off my domestic skills. I decided to bake a cake. He came over and I began my culinary show, but my very long hair got caught in the electric mixer. I remember the mixer barreling toward my head, tangling my hair in the process. I screamed bloody murder. There was cake batter everywhere, including all over my face. It was probably not one of my stronger showings in retrospect, but now it's kind of hilarious to me.

My best friend, Kerri, and I took turns being the high school mascot our senior year. Our mascot was a warrior. It was a big, ugly, offensive costume with a huge nose. There is no way that such ugliness would be acceptable today. I was young, ignorant, and naïve, and I didn't know a thing about Native American history or culture and all the injustices these people have suffered. We always wanted to be the warrior and not the Indian princess. We would debate about who got to be stuffed into the hot, sweaty costume. I am certain a lot of other people suited up in that costume, so it had years of sweat built up inside. The Indian princess was much cuter and a lot more comfortable, so I'm not sure what the appeal was to the warrior costume: maybe an opportunity to act outrageously.

I went to college in Ohio and began dating Dan, my husband-to-be. I majored in psychology and English, and

I was quite successful academically. The photograph that follows shows an academic award I won. In my senior year, I was on the homecoming court, and I took over as co-president of the Greek Council when my friend went to Belize. I was voted Greek Queen. (A nominee from each fraternity and sorority represents Greek life. It's no wonder I won; my sorority was the largest on campus.) My senior year, I was in charge of pledging for my sorority, a title we called the "pledge mistress." That role sounds like a snobby villainess from a bad eighties movie. At the time, though, my life was great. I was a big fish in a very, very small pond.

Al Hobson was a 1977 alum--a double-major in English and Communication & Theatre Arts--who died in an automobile accident a year after he graduated.

At the time of his death, friends established the Hobson Award so that, once each year, we would smile in remembrance of Al's approach to life.

Al was a good student, but what his friends and faculty recall is his wit. He enjoyed making people laugh, and he could generate hilarity by relating the simplest anecdote. Today's Hobson winner has that same ability.

Al's talents as a poet and an actor are also paralleled in this year's choice--although he would have wanted to play Snake, rather than Eve, in the recent Shaw play.

Finally, Al valued the life of the spirit, and he would be pleased to bestow his award on an ENG/PSY major who got to miss the first day of final exams by presenting a scholarly paper in Chicago!

This year's Hobson winner is Sarah Celio.

This is a photograph of the Hobson award, an honor I received in college.

Two months later Dan and I moved to Erie, Pennsylvania, where he went to medical school, we were married and we continued to live there for ten years. We rented a small bungalow with a minuscule fenced-in back yard, which was soon overflowing with two golden retrievers, Hunter and Kimble. They pretended to be lap dogs, even as they grew upward of eighty pounds each. Their favorite outing was going to the frigid waters of Presque Isle on Lake Erie, where they would barge into the icy waters for a bracing swim.

I worked as director of a life-skills program and received my master's degree in counseling, specializing in guidance counseling. The duties of my job included supervising my staff, which worked with clients facing developmental and emotional difficulties, but it was very important to me, and my agency, to continue to advocate for the people we served and to treat them with dignity. My program provided day services to people who lived in our group homes, who did not fit into traditional programs or sheltered workshops for various reasons. I loved the people I served, and I cherish the memories of them.

I started at the bottom and worked my way up. I liked that about my agency. Most of the administrative supervisors started practicing direct care, and that gave us a unique and understanding perspective. Often I worked with a very aggressive population. When I told one teenager who lived in a group home that he had probably salted his corn enough,

13

he threw a knife at my head. Yet, he remained one of my favorite people the entire time I worked there; I truly believe he was not responsible for his actions. There were days when he said, "I wish my brain wasn't like this," and that broke my heart. He loved the movie *Ghostbusters,* and when I was on his good side, I was Jeannine from the movie and could ride in his Ghostbuster car. When I was on his really good side, I could ride in the front seat.

Dan and I managed a co-ed softball team in a social service league. As a player I was always bad but, overall, the team became really good. I had a lot of fun with the team, bonding over cheese steaks and beer after the games. I remember one time throwing the ball backwards to another outfielder who had a really good arm, because I could not throw the ball all the way in from the outfield. While this move was perfectly logical to me, my teammates just thought I was throwing the ball the wrong way. I could hear howls of laughter from my teammates, and I had to giggle too because I knew how ridiculous that must have seemed.

I probably should not have picked the longest, most expensive master's program I could find, but I did. I went to Gannon University in Erie, a small, private institution. Working full time and going to school at night was difficult. It was very stressful, but I had a very encouraging boss who allowed me to adapt my busy schedule to facilitate my educational process. My professors were amazing as well. I took one class that based much of the curriculum around sensitivity training. We spent an entire class traveling around the city in a wheelchair. It was very hard. I learned about the difficulties posed by being in a wheelchair, from uneven sidewalks to inclement weather. Who knew that would become such an important lesson for me? I befriended a disabled man in a wheelchair and brought him back to class with me to tell his story.

In Erie, I began having horrible neck pains. My neck was often stiff, and I could not turn my head from side to side. My friend Karlyn had the same symptoms, so I didn't think that having neck pain was unusual. I chalked it up to stress. I have no evidence that my neck pains were related to my aneurysms, but my husband suggested the aneurysms might have been growing when I had those pains.

Education was always considered very important in my family, so when I got married at twenty-three, I made a promise to my father that I would earn an advanced degree. I *never* break a promise, and I am glad I earned that degree when I could. "My word is stronger than oak" is a quote from the movie *Jerry Maguire* and defines my beliefs perfectly. I do not break my word, because that defines my character. I have been on the receiving end of broken promises, as most of us have, and it does not feel good. I consider a broken promise to be as egregious as telling a lie. It's simple: I don't make a promise I can't keep.

My other mantras are to stay out of business that isn't mine and to always keep a secret when one is entrusted to me. I don't like drama, and disclosing secrets is a surefire way to start a conflict. I have learned not to get involved with other people's business, because that clearly causes drama. I believe confidentiality in counseling helped me learn to keep my mouth shut, which is predominantly beneficial.

We moved to east Tennessee, on the Virginia border, when my husband took a job as an orthopedic trauma surgeon. Rural Tennessee slapped me with a bit of culture shock. I was a fast-forward gal stuck in a slow-motion movie. Some folks have very thick Appalachian accents here, and the accents are quite alien to my New England staccato. One lady at my gynecologist's office said, "You should make an appointment for a yearly anal." I thought, *Boy, they are thorough here,* until I realized she meant "annual."

I was consistently surprised when people I met inevitably asked, by way of introduction, which Baptist church I attended. I am Catholic, but that denomination is not popular in the Appalachian South.

I had loved my job very much in Erie, but it was disappointing and a little insulting to me that the salary I worked so hard to earn in a year, my surgeon-husband could exceed in a month. (Today I couldn't work even if I wanted to.) To start all over accruing vacation time also seemed like a long-term nightmare.

I was officially the doctor's wife, though I often joked that I sucked at it. I watched so many women whose identities became tied to their husband's careers, and I did not like being an appendage. I was determined to keep my own identity. I rarely went to Dan's work functions, stayed out of hospital business and I was unimpressed by other people's possessions, like houses and cars. I enjoyed many perquisites of wealth- don't get me wrong - but I didn't measure my worth by our possessions. Social climbing has never been in my nature, and thankfully, my husband agreed, so he didn't seem to mind my lack of involvement.

In 2011, I became a certified ghost hunter. We were learning to communicate with spirits with a skill called "dowsing." Dowsing is achieved by using two rods to which assist in communication with spirits and can also be used to find water and ore. While we were learning that technique, the instructor asked a spirit how it arrived: the rods pointed directly at me.

I did not recognize the name of the male spirit but he said he had been with me for quite some time. Our instructor told me the spirit was adamant about giving me a warning. He said he had received only one other warning in many years of ghost hunting. It was disconcerting but I dismissed it after a few days. It makes perfect sense to me now.

I used to be very extroverted. In fact, I earned the nickname "the Party." I was given that nickname visiting some of Kevin's friends in Nashville, TN, on an impromptu bar crawl because we could not get concert tickets. I used to be quite fun. Now I am forced to be extremely introverted because I don't function well.

CHAPTER 3

The Event

I had been having terrible headaches for several weeks, which was extremely unusual for me. My friends later recalled that I had casually mentioned the headaches when I chatted with them. Aaron said we spoke on the telephone about a month before the trauma occurred, and I predicted that something terrible was going to happen. I have often been able to predict horrific events; it's just a feeling I get. I can't see the future or name specific events that are going to occur, or when an event will occur precisely, but I know when something bad is going to happen. For example, we were in Mexico and my uncle was supposed to pick us up when we landed at the airport in Florida. I told Dan as we were leaving that something terrible had happened, but I don't like to fly, so I attributed my feelings of uneasiness to that. My uncle didn't pick us up when we landed. He had a stroke while driving and was in the ICU.

I was reminded of Ellen, a girl I grew up with who died in high school. I was sitting with my best friend before I left for a dance tour in Europe, and I predicted that something terrible was going to happen while I was away. Kerri told me that I was about to have the time of my life and she didn't understand the dark feelings I was having about that trip. While our jazz band, dancers, and choir were on tour, Ellen died of an aneurysm rupture. Being a bit of a hypochondriac, I thought I had developed an aneurysm also, until I actually had my own traumatic medical event. It wasn't constantly in the forefront of my mind, but the thought was always lingering.

As it turned out, I had several aneurysms. I learned about them when one ruptured. If I had known about them earlier, it could have saved me a great deal of trouble and suffering. My aneurysms (a localized, pathological, blood-filled dilatation of a blood vessel caused by a disease or weakening of the vessel's wall) were pretty small, as far as the medical community is concerned (7.4 × 6.6 mm and 4 × 2.3 mm), so they probably would not have treated them, even if they had been detected.

The day the event occurred, I had said to my husband, "I'm going to have an aneurysm rupture." He dismissed it, and then I did. I was only thirty-seven, after all. No matter. This particular illness is nondiscriminatory concerning gender, age, race, or prior health.

The night before it all happened, we went to a birthday party and drank shots of whiskey. The next day, we celebrated my friend's actual birthday at Hooters. I had "naked" chicken wings, grilled with no breading, not deep-fried. All was right with the world.

The back cover of this book shows a picture taken the night before the monumental event happened. I was blissfully unaware that my life was about to change forever.

On March 11, 2012, at about 5:00 p.m., everything began to go awry. Our house is quite large and has several separate decks. I was on one deck, and my husband was on another, getting the good news that his high school basketball team had been inducted into the High School Hall of Fame. Birds were chirping, and suddenly, they were not. I became deaf. I now know my brain was filling with blood. When I stood up, my legs weren't working; I was able to get inside and yell to my husband for help. He called 911, thank goodness, because I couldn't have.

Dan is also in the Army Reserves, and he had received orders to be deployed that very day to Iraq. Congressman Phil Roe had worked hard to get his deployment pushed back, because Dan's hospital had just begun a residency program, and Dan played an integral part in its certification. I saw our Representative on a golf course the day before my traumatic event, and I gave him a big hug and thanked him for his hard work. Little did I realize, his hard work probably saved my life. I saw him on a commuter flight recently and it was a strange feeling to see the person solely responsible for me being alive. I thought there was no way to properly thank him, so I said nothing at all, and I am not left speechless often. I would not have survived if Dan had not been there. I would not have called 911, because I always found that going to the emergency room visits were histrionic and a waste of time. That skepticism has disappeared.

After he called the emergency number, Dan called our friend Kevin. By then I had made my way to the other deck, where my husband had been talking on the phone. I just lay on the deck and waited. I remember looking at the evening sky, flanked by my two golden retrievers standing guard, and thought, *so, this is it.* I felt the unexpected fingers of death beckoning me. I was not thinking about material things at that time; I was thinking about people I cared about and chores I had not finished. It was occasionally painful (I had neck spasms, which I later learned were most likely from my brain stem herniating), but for the most part, it was an oddly tranquil moment.

The ambulance seemed to take forever to arrive. After all, we live in a small town with no community ambulance service. Kevin got to our house before the EMTs and let them in (he lived about half an hour away). Good thing it wasn't a heart attack! I was a CPR instructor at my old job and learned that when a heart attack strikes, time is of the essence.

I was driven to the nearest hospital, about thirty minutes away, and sat on a gurney in the Emergency Room. At that moment I didn't think I had a serious problem. Ironically, we were in the same hospital where my husband operates on accident victims who have suffered terrible injuries. Someone was vomiting, and I remember thinking, *gross*. That's the final thing I remember for some time.

We had been smoking meat that day, and the last meal I had eaten was smoked chicken. I also started vomiting, and my husband said all he could smell was smoked meat. I have no recollection of getting sick to my stomach. We later gave that smoker away, and to this day, the smell of smoked meat makes both of us nauseated. We realized it for the first time some eight weeks later when Dan was wheeling me in my wheelchair from my rehabilitation center to dinner. It made us both feel sick, and I just wanted to escape that smell. There was a period of time after my trauma when I was hypersensitive to all odors. I have returned to a typical perception of scents now.

Dan knew something was terribly wrong when I regurgitated, because that was highly unusual for me. My husband, the trauma surgeon, later told me he had never seen the words "life-threatening" on a patient's bedside monitor before. He was told to call my family because I probably wasn't going to live.

It all remains a little unclear, but the neurosurgeons later told me I had two aneurysms, and one ruptured. My brain swelled to a dangerous degree and started to push through my skull and down my neck. At 3:30 a.m., a hastily summoned rescue plane flew me to University of Virginia in Charlottesville, about five hours away. That black-of-night flight, just a grim pilot, Dan and I, must have been excruciating for the conscious ones. I was comatose. UVA's Center for Neurological Injuries was the most highly regarded brain surgery facility in the region. One neurosurgeon told Dan that my age and the location of my aneurysms made my odds of survival ten million to one. It was like winning the lottery in reverse. Subsequently, I discovered that my condition was a hot topic of interest among the UVA neurosurgeons, simply because an aneurysm occurring in the brain stem region is extremely rare, particularly in a patient of my age. Their emergency treatment and its effects on my ability to function could make a fascinating article in a medical journal, said one ambitious physician.

There are two ways to treat aneurysms, clipping and coiling, and they were going to coil mine, but there was a risk of inducing a stroke, which occurred. I had a cerebellar stroke. I believe this treatment and the possible outcomes will be considered barbaric someday. The cerebellum is located in the back of the brain and controls body movement, eye movement, coordination, and balance. This stroke impacted my left side the worst. I also had vasospasms (sudden constrictions of blood vessels causing reduced blood flow or even dammed up blood flow, which are common in all brain bleeds.) During my recovery in the neuro-intensive care unit, such sudden spasms could have been fatal by themselves alone. The staff kept me under strict surveillance for four days, just five minutes from the operating room should I relapse. They shaved part of my head and put in a drain to reduce swelling (my hair has grown out since then. My friend and hairdresser, Suzanne, recently gave me bangs. She calls them "unintentional bangs." So true. I had no choice.)

I was in the intensive care unit for brain injuries/trauma for a few weeks, but I have very few memories of being there. People who have suffered from a stroke often recount that they were in a "brain fog" for some period afterwards, and I certainly was as well. The fog is finally lifting almost a year and a half later. It took me a really long time to feel remotely normal again. I remember briefly seeing my dad and stepmom who had rushed from New England to Virginia with my brother and mother. I would reach up to touch the drain in my brain, and people would hold my hands down because I incessantly attempted to pull out tubes and wires. My husband told me I would look at him devilishly as I intentionally pulled at the mechanisms monitoring my various outputs out and say, "It just fell out."

I remember my mom eating my food. Other than that, I was in a complete blur. I thought I was on the *Titanic* in Australia! A friend had recently moved to Australia, and I wanted to contact her. A nurse asked Dan if I was French, because I was speaking in French. I don't speak French. Visitors recall that I was talking to people and apparently participating in therapies, but I was a far cry from alert. I had to learn everything from scratch: going to the bathroom, sitting up, talking, walking, eating, controlling my breathing and swallowing.

The staff woke me up every hour, on the hour, for twelve days. I was given a full neurological examination, including a full battery of questions and physical demonstrations. Needless to say, I was fatigued and I wanted to be left undisturbed. I don't clearly recall, but I was told that I, and my family, didn't take well to me being poked, prodded, and mentally battered. Dan said that nurses were anxious to work with me, however. I was told that I was pretty nice and cooperative under the circumstances. Dan told me I greeted most staff with a smile. The only time I became combative was when I had to use the restroom, and no one helped me promptly, because people assumed I had maintained normal excretory control; I was not so certain.

I introduced my brother, Matt, to the nurses as my only black brother. I have no idea what that means. He is the fairest skinned of all of us, and we have the same parents; I am not black. My Caucasian family members floated through my consciousness, looking distraught but consoling, during these weeks at the UVA hospital's brain injury center.

My brother Steve said when he arrived he told me how good I looked. Apparently I responded, "Yeah. That's exactly what I'm going for right now. Looking good." I guess I looked better than in a coffin, and he was glad to hear I was maintaining a sense of humor. There may have been other lucid moments, but many more were incoherent, and my memories of those incidents are gone.

I was very concerned, apparently, about getting my pants back. For some reason, I had to see my jeans.

Kevin said he was going to feed me in the hospital one day. He pushed the tray up to me and said I was looking at him funny. As it turned out, he smashed my breasts down with the tray like a mammogram.

The nurses said I was ready to eat regular meals, so Dan asked me what I wanted. I ordered champagne cocktails, lobster, and beef Wellington. I had never had a champagne cocktail in thirty-seven years, but I am sure to order them now if I see one on a menu. I said I was tired of hospital chicken and biscuits.

I was not responsible for anything I did or said there. I simply don't remember. I could have been doing horribly mean or embarrassing things. Who knows? I now know my whole family had rushed to Virginia, along with a few friends and my husband's father. I understand that in a crisis, people want to be there, but it was wasted on me.

At one point, I was seeing angels. I wonder now if they were guardian angels or if they were angels coming to get me. At least they weren't demons.

Perhaps to allay his desperation, Dan began recording notes in a journal. Here are some of my husband's notes from two days after the event occurred. They are written frantically, therefore they are a little difficult to read, so I transcribed them immediately following in case they are illegible.

THOUGHTS ① you got mad at me.
wanted me to Do something
I couldn't. Tore me up all over.
② Trickster — How you got
the gloves off (mittens)
③ Facebook — you are lighting
up facebook with everyone posting
pictures of you with everyone.
It is so touching / amazing / heartfelt
④ I'm a Doctor but feel
helpless.. All I can do is love
you support, encourage. You
are and will always be my Rock.
⑤ First smile - 11:30
⑥ First words - 11:50 - "I know I
had a stroke"
⑦ First step 15:45 then sat in chair
⑧ First written - where's Dan
⑨ Asked to go home ⑩ smiled when
you got your phone
⑪ Asked for your pants

3/12/12- UVA

1. You got mad at me. Wanted me to do something. I
   couldn't. Tore me up all over.
2. Trickster: How you got off the gloves (mittens).

3. Face book: You are lighting up Face book with everyone posting pictures of you with everyone. It is so touching/amazing/heartfelt.

4. I'm a doctor but I feel helpless. All I can do is love you, support, encourage. You are and always will be my rock.

5. First smile: 11:30.

6. First words: 11:50: "I know I had a stroke."

7. First step: 3:48, then sat in a chair.

8. First written words: "Where's Dan?"

9. Asked to go home.

10. Smiled when you got your phone.

11. Asked for your pants.

CHAPTER 4

Inpatient Rehab

After several weeks in semiconscious limbo, I started to come to and was transferred to a brain and spinal cord injury center, where I stayed for almost a month. I hated it there. Imagine, please, your normal life gone.

I awoke to no freedom: I could not walk, I was blind, my speech was garbled, and I could not hear well. I was made to feel like I was insane and incompetent. No one believed anything I said. I felt like a prisoner in solitary confinement, yet I had done nothing wrong. My infirmities felt like prison walls. An awful, helpless feeling consumed me. I would not wish this experience on anyone.

The philosophy behind my rehabilitation regimen, designed especially for young patients, is to condition neural responses through arduous and purposefully taxing therapy sessions. It was a boot camp for battered brains. My rehab's intent was to compel derailed brain cells back onto functional tracks through the will of the patient to get better. The theory is that the damaged brain is malleable and that virtually all patient's desires to regain their health will prevail. In my case, although my senses were short-circuited and my physical coordination was malfunctioning, my capacity for rational thought and understanding was never compromised. This rare mixture of my impairments and capacities did not fit the rehabilitation paradigm, because I was not like most patients they treat. I was penned up and put on the one way, only way, hamster wheel to recovery.

I liked my speech therapist, Annie. I liked one of the nurses, Betsy, and sometimes I liked Katrina, another nurse, who plucked my eyebrows and did my hair. I liked Annie because she treated me like I had been treated before the trauma, and she did not seem to mind my problems. She was about my age and I felt that in a parallel universe, we would have been friends. We went out to lunch, and she was my confidant.

I liked Betsy for very different reasons. She was like a warden, very strict, and played by the rules. I welcomed her structure and felt certain that I would never be hurt if she was there. I breathed a sigh of relief any time I saw she was on duty. I also believed that she advocated for me as a person, and I felt that she put my needs ahead of my husband's needs, which most people did not. The nursing staff seemed more anxious to please him than to care for me.

I was grateful when Katrina did my hair in a French braid and plucked my eyebrows, because I looked and felt terrible, so unlike myself. She "rescued" me from Cassie, a nurse who was torturing me (more about that follows). She told her to leave my room when I asked for her help. Katrina also told me not to trust my husband. I did not like her then, on the Dan bashing bandwagon.

I liked my two physical therapists, Jill and Sarah, as well. They were nice to me on most occasions. I think it was Jill who ordered me to get on a machine that simulated I was falling: everything was moving around me, like a ride at a carnival. That simulator was really difficult for me; my vision was so impaired that I could only see a confusing bunch of bright colors, and my balance was terrible. But there were no options; I had to serve my time in the kaleidoscope.

I started to regain some perspective there, and it was very ugly. Finally, I began to understand the enormity of what had happened and discovered that I had lost a lot of time. I had spent nearly three weeks in the UVA hospital, but they were a blank in my memory. At my rehabilitation hospital, a group of doctors filed in every day, asked me myriad questions, and then ordered me to touch my nose and then touch their fingers. They do this to test for ataxia (the inability to coordinate voluntary body movements). I could not walk, but they claimed they found me in a chair twice (was I a miracle walker?), so I was restrained every night and whenever my husband was not present. He never saw me attempt to get out of bed, though frequently my "neighbor" wandered into my room.

I was never, ever aggressive at the rehab facility. I now realize I was frustrated enough to punch many people in the nose. I should have if I was restrained anyway and aggression was expected of me. With my blindness and poor depth perception, the chances I would have been accurate are pretty slim anyway. At my old job in Erie, the staff restrained clients only when they were a danger to themselves or others, and I never felt I was capable of any harm. I never had privacy; I was always observed going to the bathroom and showering. Dignity disappeared at the door.

I was legally blind, though no one believed me. When one is legally blind, some things can be seen poorly, so everyone assumed I could see fine when they observed me looking in the direction of objects they pointed out or reacting to noises. I could see some objects, colors, and light but no details of objects or faces. I attempted to watch television once and had to hold the monitor inches from my face and look out of the peripheral area of my right eye in an attempt to focus. I gave up quickly because that didn't work.

I was given permission to see the movie *The Hunger Games,* and I did not admit to Dan that I could not see the screen until the movie was almost over. I also had to wear audio enhancing headphones because of my hearing loss, and I tried to counteract my poor vision again by turning my head to the side and not looking at the screen directly. It did not help, but I certainly must have been a sight!

I found a video of my graduation from inpatient rehabilitation on my phone, and it was like seeing all of my therapists for the first time. I had to ask Dan who everybody was, even though I had spent hundreds of hours with those people.

I found out when I got home that I was, in fact, legally blind. It was so frustrating that no one believed me when I told everyone I could not see. A year and a half later, people continue to overrate my vision. Trust me, I have no reason to lie. When someone says my sight seems fairly well, I wish that they could see things from my perspective for just a minute. I have both double vision and blurred vision, and I can't make out anything at a distance.

During my inpatient rehab, my group therapy was doing art (a child could paint better). I made my friend a coffee mug with her initial on it. The mug was green with a purple "A," and it could hold an entire pot of coffee. She didn't even drink coffee. I played Wii bowling and located a store on a map of the mall and then found that store on a field trip, all great therapy for a blind person.

For my occupational therapy, I was dispatched to a drugstore to buy feminine hygiene products for my therapist. She wheeled me there in a wheelchair and handed me the products and cash to pay for them. Was this facility for rehabilitation also a mental hospital? Had these people heard of the book *One Flew Over the Cuckoo Cuckoo's Nest?*

CHAPTER 5

Dark Days

Within a few days I was tested to see if I could be left alone without restraints, which entailed staying in bed seventy-two hours, under observation. That is when my experience at my inpatient rehabilitation facility went from bad to absolute hell.

On April 13, 2012, during testing, two nurses were in my room, along with Dan and Kevin as I went to bed. I woke up a little while later, and they were all gone. I set off my bed alarm in order to summon someone, because I knew I should not be alone and that the nurses were supposed to be there. One of the nurses came and said the testing was over. I knew that was a lie because it was still the weekend and only my medical team could make that decision on Monday. No one on my team worked on the weekend.

Nurse Cassie came back, and she verbally tortured me for hours. She told me that my husband was cheating on me. She said she and her co-worker Lisa went to dinner with Dan and Kevin, which I later learned was untrue. I should have known that was a lie when I watched her introduce herself to my husband the next morning. Lisa seemed poised to come in but just stood in the doorway, crying. She slipped away that night and never returned.

Of course, I tried to call my husband but could not see the phone dial pad, so it was nearly impossible to dial numbers correctly. Finally, I was able to dial his number by feeling the keypad; of course, the nurses had been lying about his infidelity. He said he had been watching me on a TV monitor outside my room and had not been allowed to enter during the testing.

Katrina came in, and I told her that I would not go to sleep until Cassie, who was tormenting me, was banished. Dan's notes show that I was sitting up, which was very unusual for me. I went to bed early on most nights there. I was sitting up because the nurse was maliciously talking to me, and I refused to go to sleep with her there. Cassie finally left, temporarily, and Katrina replaced her.

Katrina, whom I liked, told me that she was working on a research paper (to which I offered to contribute) and told me not to trust my husband (I called her sometime after I had returned home and confronted her, but she denied my allegations, though she did acknowledge that Cassie had been lying to me). I woke up to her sneaking out on me, too. That was typical. I was not supposed to be left alone, but I often was. That was fine with me.

Cassie kept returning; the next morning, she showered in my bathroom to get ready for her day. Nice. That nurse thoroughly scared me; I thought she was going to hurt me, and she didn't appear to be mentally stable. She would bounce from saying horrible things to saying, "I like you so much." It made no sense. She gave me the creeps, and the thought of her watching me while I slept did not help.

Lisa came back the next day to help me with my personal hygiene; I thought, *No way is she seeing me naked*. She said very sincerely, "Sorry for ruining your life, Sarah."

I told everyone I trusted about this incident, but no one could tell me how to file a complaint. When I did file a complaint, a year later, the facility's administrator never even contacted me personally, but wrote a letter to my husband, basically saying I remembered everything wrong; my chart even said so. I remember every detail about that night, including names (which I have changed to protect the identities of the people I didn't care for). No one ever asked me the details. It would have been very useful to speak to me. I do not even know what it was they thought they were investigating.

Dan was my guardian during my rehabilitation. His presence, I must conclude, saved me from worse treatment. When he did rarely leave, he utilized the family living quarters (apartments) at my rehabilitation center and remained close by, from the night of my catastrophe until I was released from rehab. Kevin was there a good deal of time as well. I slept erratically and often found myself entirely alone or under scrutiny from staff members I could not trust.

I was physically drained and mentally fatigued because my traumatized brain cells craved rest. At one point, a day nurse grabbed my face and squeezed my cheeks to quell my protests and told me I couldn't go back to bed between therapies. I spun around in my wheelchair and propelled myself to the nurses' station to complain, but my a nurse retorted, "We have a love/hate relationship." I told the duty station nurse/supervisor, "No, it's just hate."

Afterwards my nurse sneered, "No one will believe you anyway," or something to that effect. Thank goodness my husband made sure she never worked with me again.

Another day, when I asked for Twizzler's, one caretaker told me I needed a man. Huh? I just wanted licorice. On a side note, I could have cared less about sweets before my attack, but I have subsequently developed a craving for them. When I got home, I devoured a carload of cupcakes. I also used to love salt. Now I am overpowered when any food is a little bit salty. I have no idea why these phenomena have occurred or why my taste buds have changed.

On yet another day, the staff was preparing to administer a battery of standardized tests. I remember saying to my husband, "If they are visual, I'm screwed," because I realized my eyes could not focus and even my peripheral perception was foggy, as if I were peering out from a fish tank. They were all visual, so, needless to say, I failed. It's not in my nature to accept any poor performance, so that was a really frustrating day. The most maddening moment was when the doctor in training called me down to evaluate my test results and then turned me away because my husband was not there. Dan is a doctor, yes, but they were *my* results! This resident's condescending behavior sent the horrible signal that I was too debilitated to understand the results. I mean, come on, people! We are stroke patients. We aren't stupid! I recently watched a documentary about a girl who suffered an injury similar to mine. When she awoke, she could not speak, but she typed over and over, "I'm the same inside." I thought that spoke volumes.

I have heard of people who have survived brain trauma being treated like imbeciles; obviously, it is infuriating. I just wanted to know if my test scores affected my escape from this incarceration. They did not. So while this treatment made me irate, I brushed it off because all I wanted was to get away from that place and go home. These affronts were very common at the rehabilitation facility.

I had no basic freedom. I was in a lockdown unit (the doors were locked so I could not escape). My wrists were manacled every night for the first few weeks so I was forced to request unshackling before I got out of bed. I had to ask permission to go outside and to sit in the sunlight. Decisions about my life were made by my team (the only people I know for sure who were members of this team were my therapists and a doctor). I was under observation during all personal hygiene activities, like showering and going to the restroom. I was told how to speak and not to swear. All of my behaviors were monitored and recorded (apparently inaccurately, if one believes the letter from the center's administration which Dan received), and they became part of my evaluation and key to my release and freedom. I cannot stress enough the frustration I felt at my rehabilitation facility.

Trust me, the way to rehabilitate a sick person is not to take away all control and choices, except for some meals. If I attempted to exert any independence, I felt stifled and punished. Any facility is only as good as it's staff. I believe that if the staff had made me feel human and good about myself, the facility would have exceeded its good reputation.

It is difficult to explain, but I am rather inflexible when it comes to what little I can control. I had not been told what to do since childhood. I am an adult now and gradually regaining greater independence. I still become very frustrated when I am told what to do or how I should feel. Over eighteen months later, in fact, I may still be reacting to the disempowerment I suffered in "rehab." Is there a feminine equivalent to emasculation? If so, I lived it.

All daily activities, from mealtimes to a carousel of rehabilitations, were strictly scheduled and written on a board in the main lobby area, to be checked every day. I walked with the help of a machine that tracked my gait; it would stop if my steps slipped out of synch. It never stopped when I was on it, and my husband thought that machine was very cool. For the most part, I just did mundane things like practicing walking and speaking articulately. For practice, Annie had me call a Blockbuster store and ask if they had the movie *What About Bob?* The man who answered could understand me; I thought that was very clever. I thought it was hilarious to prank call people for therapy.

When I think back to my time at my rehabilitation facility, I remember two kinds of days: bad days and really bad days. On really bad days, look out world! If I felt my friends and family failed to defend me, they would hear about it in a not-so-nice way. I have a great deal of resentment because everyone I thought would protect me seemed to have abandoned me in my rehabilitation facility, even though I was persistently telling people about my mistreatment. Unfortunately, the ones nearest and most beloved to me are often the targets of my frustration. All of the people with whom I discussed it have told me they believed they were taking the best course to speed my recovery. My caretakers acquiesced to my appearances, succumbed the temptations of perceiving my obvious impairments as an accurate rendition of my entire perception of my personality, and ignored my cognitive abilities, which I could only express with great labor.

I *begged* everyone I loved to help me get out of there. No one did. I was helpless, and no one seemed to care. I was made to feel stupid and crazy. I had to watch as my visitors politely engaged with the very people who were so cruel to me. I later learned that three of my girlfriends had come to visit me but weren't allowed in; yet my friend's ex-boyfriend, whom I met only once briefly, was allowed into my room. That makes zero sense. I even threatened to drive myself away from the hospital, if any visitor would offer me some car keys, and I was blind! It is testimony to how distraught I felt.

I asked a doctor if I could stay at a hotel and continue to do therapy, and he told me it didn't work that way. It was all or nothing.

My brother and his wife came to visit me, and I was certain they would take me away from there when they learned of my treatment. I even packed my suitcase because I was so certain they would take me anywhere but the facility. They didn't save me. Everyone believed I was getting the treatment I needed. I recently talked to my sister-in-law, Tiffany, and she said I pleaded with her, asking what she would do if her own daughter was being mistreated. She responded with empathy but made no move to extricate me. At least I could still appeal to people logically and on a relatable level.

On the upside, the food at the inpatient rehabilitation hospital was terrific.

I had about seven hours of therapy a day at the facility: physical therapy, speech therapy, occupational therapy, and group therapy. I felt like it didn't help much, but progress is *very* slow with a cerebellar stroke. When I left, I could use a walker, rather than only a wheelchair, so that was considerable progress. Some time later, I found a video on my phone. My speech was so bad that I could not understand myself. I think I said, "Say hi to Dan," to Dan. Whom did I think I was telling that to? I give my speech therapist and husband an immense amount of credit. I'm sure that my disabilities were as frustrating for them as they were for me.

During my illness and stay at the rehabilitation facility, I hit a low of 103 pounds (I am five feet five inches tall). I recall my jeans literally falling off of my body during therapy. My husband said I had a perpetual plumber's crack. It was probably a combination of being so sick, stress, not drinking alcohol, and a fast metabolism. I drank Ensure to keep my weight at a healthy level. I am so thankful for that genetic make-up now, because I am fairly sedentary compared to what I was before the trauma. I haven't gained a lot of weight but I have definitely lost muscle mass and tone. It was kind of scary, because I wasn't trying to lose weight, yet I was wasting away. I was a gym fanatic before (personal trainer, endless boot camps), but that has all ceased because I still walk unsteadily. The boot camp at my rehab was more rigorous but not half as invigorating as regular exercise. It was all work at rehab: no music, socialization, or fun. I am not afraid of hard work. I recognize therapy and recovery is not a day at the beach.

My personal trainer, Cody, might tell you that I was disciplined and a hard worker. He might also tell you that I had to leave a few training sessions early in the days leading up to my traumatic event. That didn't happen often but I felt dizzy and under the weather on the days I escaped prematurely. At my best, I was in the ninety-eighth percentile of body fat for my age. I believe that being in strong physical condition going into my event helped me survive.

When another sister-in-law came to visit, it was a comedy of errors. We get along well. In fact, she was the matron of honor in my wedding. We took a trip to the mall, and she tripped on a curb and fell. It was ironic, because I was the one who could not see. She also made me go "commando" when my husband went home. She said I didn't have enough underwear to last the week. Dan said I called him and complained that she was making me go without underwear. We still laugh about that to this day. When I was discharged from the hospital, we went to a spa and got facials. She told me to take my pants off. I asked her, "For a facial?"

I go to the spa a lot now for relaxation. I like it there very much because it is calming and the people are so nice. The first time I went after my stay at my rehabilitation facility, they refused to give me a massage. I felt like enough of an outcast already. That did not help matters.

I have had many people say that chapter of my life is over, and I have been advised to let it go, but I can't. When you are so helpless and abused during a critical time, it leaves a scar on your psyche. I had no control of any part of my life. When you are sick, you are supposed to be nurtured, cared for, and protected by nurses and loved ones, not tortured. That's exactly what happened, and no one believed me. Who knows how long my anger about the way I was treated will last, but it remains a travesty in my mind. I am still very angry and frustrated with so many people. I had conducted investigations of mistreatment by caregivers (among other investigations) as part of my life skills director job in Erie, and I am acutely aware that everything was poorly handled.

CHAPTER 6

The Investigation Results

About a year later, I filed a complaint and the facility conducted an investigation. There was no action taken against the staff. I originally included a copy of the investigation results but upon legal advice I have rewritten parts of their letter in my own words and added my responses, to illustrate the callousness to which I have grown accustomed. The letter was sent to my husband, not to me.

First, the letter begins with an apology that we had to file a complaint about my treatment. Were they sorry I was treated that way or sorry I filed a complaint?

Second, since my allegations were made almost a year after I was released, they would be difficult to substantiate. Again, I was never told that there was a time limit for filing a complaint. If anyone had told me, I certainly would have filed a complaint more promptly.

Third, they claimed they interviewed the majority of the staff that was related to my stay. I wonder why everyone wasn't interviewed. I am not quite sure what the interviews entailed, because no one ever contacted me about this investigation, nor were the contents of those interviews disclosed.

Fourth, the letter said that there was no documentation concerning the alleged verbal abuse by their nurses nor were there any staff who could remember these complaints coming up during my stay or had any knowledge of the alleged complaint. Who would document verbal abuse? No one would enter in his or her notes, "I gave Sarah her medication and then I verbally abused her for a while." I am very disappointed that the people I told about this incident pretended they had no knowledge about these events. They do. Maybe they just did not understand my unintelligible speech, at the time.

Fifth, the letter stated that several staff members have been noted for exemplary customer service. It is not my fault that they turned a blind eye to improper treatment. I am just stating the truth. My experience, exactly the way it happened, is indelible on my mind. It has no relation to any awards received by some staffers.

Sixth, the letter indicated that a traumatic brain injury could cause cognitive difficulties, in which things could be perceived in an inaccurate way; my records showed that I was exhibiting a lack of "insight." I am certain that my accounts, and related details, are accurate. There were times when my recollection was inaccurate, and I can admit when I was not mentally clear. Everything about their uncaring behavior is seared into my memory on the crucial night in question.

Of course my chart said I was confused. Who composed the chart? All the conspirators who worked there were erasing their tracks. All my problems were overwhelmingly physical, not cognitive.

Here are Dan's notes from the night I claimed the nurses were so horrible to me. I again have transcribed them immediately after his notes to make them easily legible.

4/13/12. Rehab facility

- Called for 4th time. Mad at us.
- I hate this. Sitting at nurse's station watching you. Why, why, why? Dr. _____ said, "no". Go sleep at Woodruff apartments.
- Sat for hours watching you sit up as the nurses, _____ and aides and watchers, sit with you. You are sitting up waiting for me.
- I hate this. I can't watch. It hurts so bad. Why can't I just sit with you? It tears me up to watch you call me, waiting. I don't care what Dr. _____ says. This isn't easy for her (Sarah) or me. Torture. I'm crying at the nurse's station and they won't let me go in.
- Kevin is outside. I have been here for 4 hours, writing. Sarah is finally asleep. It is 2 a.m. I am going to try to sleep and then be back at 6 a.m. for her and P.T./shower. Love her more than life.

I have heard quite a few cerebellar stroke victims say the same thing: inside the patient's head thoughts are coming fast and normally, but no one responds because of the blatantly visible symptoms of stroke – the bandaged skull, the stent draining brain fluids, the distended facial muscles, the staples in the shaved head, slurred speech and the vague and glazed eye contact – overwhelm observers. That phenomenon of disconnection between the patient's mind and body, and the unanticipated, incorrect responses cause a great deal of frustration.

What kind of people taunts a sick patient for entertainment, anyway? What was their intention? To break me down? They did. They informed me I had to repeat the test to overcome restraints because I had *sat up* once. Does 150 hours in bed seem an absurd penance because a patient sits up? You bet. I believe no one who works with stroke patients fully understands what it is like to survive this trauma; one must experience it personally. I talked to a lovely man I apparently met at my inpatient therapy (my blindness precluded me from recognizing him), and he claimed he had a very positive experience in the same hospital. I believe they counted on me not recollecting properly and I believe some people do not.

I never completed the second test, because Dan signed paperwork saying that I did not have to be restrained. The papers absolved the responsibility of the rehabilitation facility if I got out of bed and got hurt. I was certain I would not get out of bed. The only time I jumped out of bed was toward the end of my stay. There was a wrapper in my bed, but because of my poor eyesight, I thought it was a cockroach. A silver cockroach. I leapt from my bed and, thankfully, landed in my wheelchair. My sister-in-law was visiting, and I remember her and my husband looking at me like I was nuts.

CHAPTER 7

Going Home

Needless to say, I was thrilled to leave the rehabilitation facility, to go home and see my dogs. My beautiful friends and my husband arranged a great homecoming. My friend Jill did all of my spring planting for me. Dan recruited my friend Erica to put flowers all over the house, and there were huge balloons waiting for me. It was a great day. My mom came and stayed for weeks. Don't get me wrong; I was very thankful for her help. She was relatively easy to have around. She cooked comfort foods for me upon my request, like meatloaf and mashed potatoes. She drove me to my therapy appointments and waited there for three hours. We tried to play cards, but my poor eyesight made that difficult. She also told my friend that I "raced up and down the stairs." That simply was not true. I *still* do not go up and down stairs quickly. People's enhancements on experiences in order to "keep the message positive" made me feel crazy. I had enough of that in the hospital.

I told her to leave after about five weeks. I just wanted to be alone. I had no privacy for months. Do not take my need for privacy as an affront. It had nothing to do with her personally. In fact, I speak to her on the telephone almost every single day. We have a good relationship.

After I got home, it was a whirlwind of doctors' appointments, surgeries, brain scans, and sensory tests. The surgeries were mostly on my eyes. My retinal surgeon was a miracle worker. He took me from blindness to some sight overnight. I went from having no surgeries in my lifetime to over a dozen in one year. At one appointment, I had to complete a standard eye exam; I covered one eye with a mask and had to read the letters on a sign. The staff said I looked like a dog, the way I cocked my head and tried to get a view of the blurry letters. I laughed along with the staff members. I know they meant no harm by that comment; in fact, I was there so often that they became very familiar to me. They always commented on the shoes I was wearing. In hindsight, I probably would not recommend comparing a patient to a dog.

Three times a week, I went to outpatient therapy at Bristol Regional Medical Center (still physical therapy, occupational therapy, and speech therapy). I did quite a bit of walking, talking, and balance-strengthening activities. Nintendo DS has two very helpful games: one for brain exercises and one for vision improvement. Wii Fit is also great for balancing activities, and it's fun! My therapists taught me how to walk with a cane. I would most likely have continued therapy if I didn't have to rely on other people for rides. That was a drain on me emotionally. Since I was exhausted and frustrated already, doctors and therapy were an added burden. I believed if I saw one more doctor, I would go into sensory overload. Very few accomplished anything, anyway.

The surgeries were on my retinas to drain the blood in my eyes from the ruptured aneurysms and to laser a hole in my macula. I had to have cataract surgery on my left eye as a result of all my retinal surgeries. Although I was out cold most of the time from anesthesia, there were two occasions when I was alert enough to feel the procedures and see a needle in my eye. On two occasions, my eye bloodied up after the surgery, and that took weeks to dissipate. It looked like I had been punched in the eye and broke some blood vessels. It wasn't painful but it looked terrible. After most of the surgeries, I had to wear a patch over my left eye for a day. I looked like a pirate.

I requested an anesthesiologist Dan knew because I didn't want to remember any more surgeries. I shook my finger at him and said, "I'm not going to remember this, am I?" I didn't. I was so thirsty because on the eves of my surgeries I couldn't eat or drink anything after midnight; I said I would drink out of a pig trough if I could find one. Unfortunately, the hospital walls were not lined with water-filled pig troughs. Afterward, my husband recounted, two of my girlfriends were talking to me, and I fell asleep as they were speaking mid-sentence. After the surgery was over, I importuned the anesthesiologist about when we were going to get the procedure started.

The surgeries were no fun, but a necessary evil. One day before the attack, I had perfect vision, and then the next day, I was blind. The loss was not a gradual degeneration. I had no time to prepare or adjust. The shock itself was paralyzing, but I was willing to try anything to restore my vision. Today, my sight is still not good, and it is impeding my walking progress and balance. My eyes do not work together, so everything seems blurry and double. One doctor said that my eyes drift and do not focus on an object. My depth perception is terrible, and I especially can't see things at a distance but it is greatly improved from my time in the rehabilitation center. Next I am to try lasering (on my cataracts), and I am seeing a neuro-ophthalmologist in Nashville. I hope it helps.

I loved all my therapists at the regional rehabilitation facility, but I hated therapy. Again, exhaustion was a real issue. No one wants to be in therapy at thirty-seven years old, three times a week, for three hours a day. That is how often I was going to physical therapy, speech therapy, and occupational therapy. No one ever wants to be in therapy, at any age. With cerebellar strokes, the energy commitment was particularly taxing, and recovery occupied most of my thoughts. Rehabilitation from a cerebellar stroke takes a great deal of time. Time became a four-letter curse word for me. One of my physical therapists told me that often with this type of neurological injury, patients do not see much progress from therapy sessions, not quickly at least. For other people, therapy can be very helpful.

Doggedly, I continued therapy for over a year, with very small victories. The people and families whom I encountered in therapy were cheerful and optimistic. We were all so different (some were in wheelchairs, some were non-verbal, some were kids, some were young adults, and some were elderly adults). Did you know a stroke could occur in the womb? I didn't. I realized it could have been so much worse, yet it was very frustrating to watch those who made faster progress, although I was genuinely happy for their victories.

The waiting room resonated with war stories: car accidents, domestic abuse, and spontaneous life changes. Everyone told unique stories, but there were lessons to be learned. For instance, I emulated one man who refused to sit on a plastic chair when he showered. I tossed my little bench from my shower stall at home. To stand up unaided during a hot shower is a small step forward, but to me it was terribly important, and I reveled in my tiny taste of independence.

Speaking of war stories, my theme song became "One" by Metallica. I could relate to everything (except the war imagery). It is a depressing song but so relatable. Now I listen to more positive music to try to remain upbeat and optimistic. I have included a list of one motivational mix I made:

"Jump Rope," Blue October
"Then I'll Be Smiling," Matt Nathanson
"Twilight," Michelle Branch

"Survivor," Destiny's Child

"Vindicated," Dashboard Confessionals

"What You Wish For," Guster

"When You Come Back Down," Nickel Creek

"Stronger," Kanye West

"Please, Please, Please, Let Me Get What I Want," The Smiths

"Just Stand Up," Various Artists

"Your Hands," JJ Heller

"Glad to Have a Friend Like You," Marlo Thomas

"The Day that I Die," The Benjy Davis Project

"The Battle," Missy Higgins

"You Gotta Be," Des'ree

"Stronger," Brittany Spears

Music was a huge part of my life before my aneurysms and stroke, so I continue to believe if you find valuable meaning in a song, let your affections stand, without judgment. Also, I can keep up with fast lyrics in my head. I definitely can't sing along with quick lyrics out loud.

CHAPTER 8

Friends

One good thing about my traumatic time: I have learned who my friends truly are. Let me give you a hint: I have fewer true friends than I thought. A person I knew who lost multiple children once gave me some wise advice: people don't need a great deal of support immediately after a tragedy (it's overwhelming when everyone is around while one is grieving). It is one, five, ten years afterwards that matters, because everyone has disappeared by then. Great advice, and that has been my experience exactly. The same person who gave me that advice never checked on me once.

At my rehabilitation facility, I was inundated with a huge outpouring of love and support. I received cards, candy, flowers, visitors, food, and gifts. I even got tons of homemade meals from people I had never even met, because another friend told people I was in the hospital in a city foreign to me. She never took credit for that, but it was really sweet.

I received a lot of photographs. My dear friend Hope made several collages of our good times, which were abundant (the staff thought she was my sister). My friends Erica, Suzanne, Brandon, Andy, and his kids made me sweet get-well packages. It was great, but that stopped, for the most part, when I got home.

Don't get me wrong, there were many who were wonderful and still are. You know who you are. My friend Konni *still* cooks for me every Thursday. That is an extraordinary contribution. That is so helpful and thoughtful.

There were also many people who ran for the hills at the first sign of adversity, people who did little or nothing. You also know who you are. I figured the unsupportive people fall into one of three categories: a) they think I have fully recovered (I have not), b) the trauma is too much to wrap their heads around, c) they are too self-centered to care. Whatever the reason is, if you were not there in my crucial time, you never will be.

My best friend, Kerri, lives in California now, and she left her two beautiful daughters and husband to visit me three months after my ruptured aneurysm and stroke. If she was startled to see me unable to walk without the assistance of a walker, she didn't show it. She bedazzled my walker with blue and green rhinestone stickers. For Halloween, my favorite holiday, I put cobwebs on my walker. I have a whole closet dedicated to costumes, from which I carefully selected a vampire costume to attend a Halloween party at Andy and Erica's home. The costume is my camouflage.

For Christmas, Dan festooned my walker with battery-powered colored lights, a garland and ornaments. The picture below includes my decorated walker and my friend, Kevin, at our Christmas celebration.

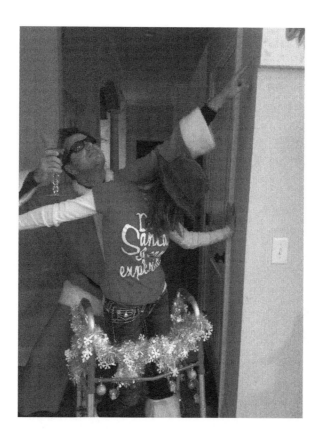

Dan and Kevin surprised me with a trip to Sun Valley, Idaho, and a rendezvous with Kerri to mark my one-year "anniversary." She bejeweled my cane, as she had done to my walker. As long as I was stuck using those implements to get around, they might as well be as fun as they could be. People at my therapy hospital loved it.

I had an eight-month string of visitors until November of 2012, and then I had none, by choice. Visitors could be exhausting. I don't know how to be anything but an attentive hostess. I cook, clean, give gifts, and pour unlimited drinks. Many people said they were coming to help. Most people did not.

During one visit in November, my husband was scheduled to work the next day. Someone I considered very wise and valued as a close friend said, "I will babysit her tomorrow." That was a big no-no. I had been alone and independent for some time. She made me feel like a child. It was very insulting. I was fortunate with this kind of stroke that I never lost my thinking speed, my mental acuity, or my sense of identity. I may have appeared diminished, but I was still as intelligent as ever.

I cursed at my friend who made me feel like an infant. Oh, by the way, people who have endured certain strokes can swear *a lot*, even if that's not normal for them. Some people also become physically combative. I never did, but at my rehabilitation facility, people often became aggressive and had to be restrained. I was clueless; blindness and deafness were a benefit in these moments.

A short time after my "helping" friends left, I received a text from another friend, asking about my progress. My husband and I had pleaded with our guests not to discuss my condition or progress with anyone. It is my story to tell, and I was not ready to tell it then. Most people think I suffered a stroke. I didn't. It is so problematic to me when my story isn't even shared accurately. I was given a stroke as a parting gift on the game show of life when trying to survive the ruptured aneurysm. Not wanting to jump to conclusions, I had asked the texting friend how he had learned about my progress. He confirmed what I had feared, naming my two friends who had just visited us.

As I often say, I appear to be a shell of the person I once was. Stroke victims just want to be treated normally, the way they were always treated. People new in my life do not know how I behaved and functioned before. I am very self-conscious about my voice. I have no desire to meet new people or see anyone I don't know well.

My speech was not totally debilitated; I never completely lost the ability to speak. Some people do. Can you imagine waking up and having no voice? That would be awful. Some people have memory loss. That would be awful as well.

My penchant for swearing has died down considerably, thank goodness. People with strokes can blurt out cruel comments and not mean them. That is so important for caretakers to understand. The victims are not angry specifically with the individual who bears the brunt of spontaneous hostility; they are frustrated and their brains are rewiring, so people around them must be patient, forgiving, and compassionate.

I was, and am, adamant that people who visit me in my home respect my privacy. That didn't happen with those friends; I asked them not to share my personal story and progress, and they did anyway.

Another friend asked if she could come for a visit and I said "No." I wasn't ready to have visitors (and I am still not).

She said, "You can't hide forever."

I responded, "I'm not hiding; I am recovering."

Her comment really upset me. People should consider the vulnerability of the recovering stroke patient before saying something like that. It was not kind or helpful. I like my friend very much; I just believe that she didn't think before she made that comment. I didn't find it humorous or cute.

I learned what it means to be a great friend through my own great friends (Dan, Kevin, Jill, Tacie, Michelle, Stephanie, Kerri, Scott, Lisa). I am sorry for the times when people were suffering and I was not more sympathetic. That will gradually change now, since experiencing my own trauma, I have developed much more sympathy toward the trials that others are enduring, especially people who are going through a traumatic experience.

Lisa is a dear friend of mine who underwent multiple surgeries on her foot. She was a runner, so I am certain that her injury was devastating for her. I do not feel like I was a good enough friend during her traumatic time. Now I would ask her what could be done that would be helpful to her, whether it be cooking, cleaning, or watering plants. Anyway, I find it more rewarding to help someone than to be helped by others.

CHAPTER 9

Invisible

My voice began to regress after November. My speech became very slow, throaty, and quiet. It was taxing to talk, and I don't recall it being so effortful before, except from a supine position. It was hard to breathe, talk, and be understood at first. The only people I talk to on the telephone are my parents (and occasionally my brothers). Thus, the feelings of isolation are exacerbated. Phone conversations are particularly burdensome. Listeners often misunderstand me or ask for numerous repetitions, and I am left feeling stifled.

Dan often has to translate for me in public. People would rather ignore a stroke victim than concentrate and try to understand. It annoys me when people talk to him as if I am not there, and that happens *a lot*. With reduced conversation and fewer interpersonal exchanges, I face extreme frustration. I feel invisible because if I do not speak, people act as if I am mentally vacant. I even asked Dan if I was already dead, because it felt as though no one could hear me.

I never order at restaurants. Heck, I rarely go out to eat.

I have lost all ability to sing. I was never a great singer, but I did act in some plays and sing some solos in Community Theater, so I was a performer who has left the stage empty. The photograph that follows is from *Leader of the Pack*, a show in which I sang the title song, among a few other songs. I cannot even whistle now. As a baby, I could whistle before I could speak, which visitors found quite amazing. Now I cannot whistle at all: a small loss, magnified. It is as if my vocal cords do not work properly. I also can't roll r's on my tongue anymore. I speak some Spanish, and that is a skill I had mastered when speaking that language, but it's gone.

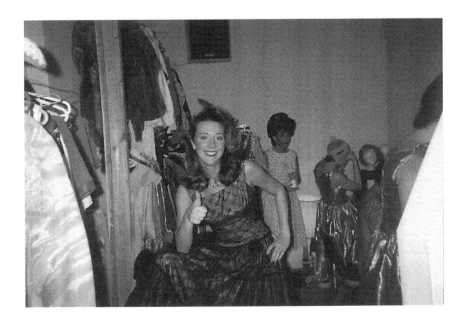

I do not hear well and constantly have a ringing in my left ear. I cannot hear people at all on the telephone if I listen with my left ear. I do not understand the source of many noises. When there are multiple noises at once, which includes multiple people talking, it is overwhelming to me. All I hear is incomprehensible noise. It is a challenge to filter out one conversation among several simultaneous chats. No more cocktail parties. Background noise is very loud, distracting, and disconcerting. It sounds like I am underwater. I can hear sounds, even loudly, but the sounds are garbled. Women's voices, or noises in a higher register, are also more difficult to hear. I had audiology testing, but they could not see any problem with my left ear or explain my hearing loss, so I guess I just have to learn to live with it. My attempts to compensate by turning my better ear toward a speaker have been construed as an inability to concentrate, when actually I am trying very hard to focus and understand.

I have an unusually high tolerance for physical pain. I made it through this whole ordeal without taking heavy-duty pain medications. I took mostly aspirin for pain management, but only infrequently. The doctors speculated that I would have terrible headaches after my trauma, but I didn't. The doctors also said I might sleep for up to seventeen hours a day upon returning home from rehabilitation, but I didn't. Sometimes sleep seems like a peaceful way to escape my problems.

CHAPTER 10

Tremors

Eating is difficult for me. I developed horrible tremors in my hands about six months post-stroke. My neurosurgeon said it is from blood settling on my spinal cord. There are not any medications to help this phenomenon, but it should improve over time. Any fine motor activity is very confounding (buttons, writing, zippers, make-up, tweezing). If I pour half a cup of coffee, I am okay. If the cup is full, I will spill it. I am very self-conscious of my tremors and do not like to eat in front of anyone as a result. They make even a tiny task that was easy for me before my trauma very difficult, like typing this story.

Fortunately, I can laugh at myself. When I spill something or look at my handwriting, it is kind of funny. Feeding my dogs is hilarious, but I can see progress. Initially when I fed them or gave them water, food and drink were scattered everywhere. Now only a few pieces of dry food spill on the floor. I am sure they miss me clumsily dropping food everywhere. They were always there eating up very delicious morsels I spilled, and they were quite pleased to clean up my messes.

At the rehabilitation facility, I used to French braid my hair every day (sloppily, I'm sure). Now, I can't do that because of the tremors in my hands. I just end up pulling my hair.

Here is an example of my writing before and after:

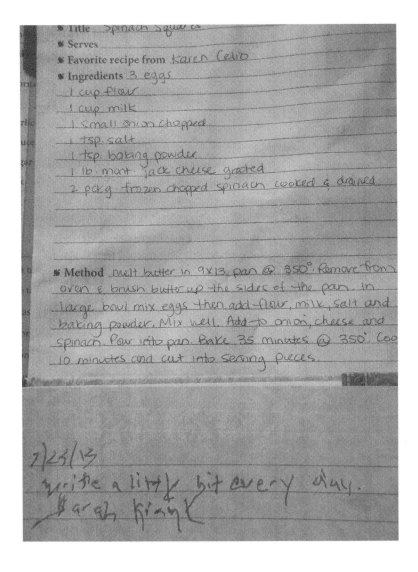

One of my friends, who is also a doctor, told me to write a little bit every day, so that is what I write. She gave me a book to record my progress, but my puppy ate it: my version of the dog ate my homework. I sometimes write the number 2 pretty well. I am thirty-eight and happy when a 2 is written well? That is sad and silly.

I attempted to make stuffed mushrooms recently. There was filling everywhere. They were so ugly that I sent a picture to my friend. They tasted the same as usual, even if it was difficult to stuff the mushrooms. Truth is in the tasting.

CHAPTER 11

Tears and Travels

I recently went on a trip to Miami with my awesome friend, Stephanie. She has some personal experiences with strokes, and she has been very understanding. I met Stephanie at Hope's wedding; we were both in the wedding party, and I am so glad we connected, because my life is richer with her in it. While we were vacationing, the waiter refused to serve me a glass of wine, because he assumed I was already hammered (the picture on this book's front cover is from that day). Stephanie had just treated me to my first hair blowout, and we went directly to the Fontainebleau Hotel for dinner. I looked normal but walked and talked as if I had been drinking. In fact, I *feel* drunk and uncoordinated much of the time. How embarrassing for me, and the waiter.

I heard Stephanie say, "No, no, no. She had a recent brain injury. You should educate yourself before jumping to conclusions."

That was the second time she had to defend me in Miami against my false drunken conduct. The first time we were out to dinner, and I took off my shoes. It's hard for me to walk in the first place, but throw in a nice pair of shoes, as appropriate for trendy South Beach, and forget it. A lady made a rude comment, and Stephanie growled stinging words at her. I didn't even hear the woman say a word.

That unthinking waiter *almost* made me cry. I lost the ability to cry when the aneurysm/stroke struck. I have a pervasively flat affect now. It feels very unnatural to smile for photos, so I force myself to take pictures every day. I am going for a Guinness world record for wearing different headgear on consecutive days, which is being chronicled in my photographs.

I found that sand poses unique problems. The ever-changing ground beneath my feet was very problematic for me. I have difficulty balancing anyhow but the perceived instability of sand is very difficult to walk upon.

I could not laugh for a long time, but now I can. It sounds different from my "old" laugh, but I can. My personality is intact, but only a few people take the time to comprehend. My husband might tell you I'm very funny. Other people with strokes say they cry all the time, so that is another thing that is variable for everyone. I am looking forward to crying again. I've had so much emotion pent up. I have experienced unthinkable sadness and frustration, but if I had to choose tears or laughter, I would choose laughter.

Flying for the first time was terrifying for me, even though I had been cleared to fly by my neurosurgeon. When I was airlifted to the University of Virginia, they had to fly under a certain altitude, because the pressure at a high altitude was perilous for my brain. Commercial airlines fly at a much higher altitude than medical emergency flights, and I just wasn't sure what flying would to do to me. That's why we chose Miami. I wanted to have US hospitals nearby just in case. A relapse always lingers in the back of my mind, and makes TBI victims worry.

I have traveled internationally a few times, and customs is a breeze now, because they push my wheelchair to the front of the line. In accommodating the needs people with disabilities, airlines and airports have demonstrated an empathy, which I appreciate immensely. In fact, I am currently editing this portion of my story from Tuscany. It's beautiful here. There are expansive valleys, and I can see for miles and hear thunder from far away, even if it is sunny. We are staying at a beautiful, three-hundred-year-old villa with a pool, a guest cottage, and outdoor pizza ovens. We watch the sun melt into the horizon every night, and I am thankful I'm alive to see another sunset.

My dad flew my entire family, sixteen people, to Italy for a month. How generous of him. I thought the trip would be overwhelming for me, but my nieces and nephews are wonderful. My niece did my hair in a fishbone braid one day, and another picked out my dresses for evening dinners. I could tell they were all trying very hard to understand my lethargic speech. My father, stepmother, siblings, and all of their wives have been very accommodating and understanding of my limitations.

I joke that I am the worst tourist ever. I can't see, hear, walk, or talk well. People told me to take a lot of pictures. Of course I will, just to see it for myself someday.

As we boarded our returning flight from Costa Rica, I overheard a man who became frustrated because I was allowed to skip ahead of him in line. It hurt my feelings immensely. I am sorry I pose an inconvenience. Trust me, anyone who is disabled would much prefer to stand in a line in order to not deal with any complications or disabilities.

In June of 2012, my dog Kimble died; she was fourteen and a half years old. I didn't cry even then, although I was extremely sad. I believe she "waited" for me to get home from rehab, to make sure I was okay. I think that pets are so important to recovery, if the patient is an animal person. I still have my other golden retriever, Hunter, though he is clearly failing of old age, too. He is such a sweet dog, and I will be heartbroken when something happens to him.

In March, we adopted/rescued a longhaired, liver-colored German shepherd; we named her Harlow. She keeps me talking and playing ball with her, and she certainly keeps me on my toes when I am walking, so that's all good for me. She is so amusing; she cocks her head as if she understands every word I say when I am speaking. That is more than I can say about most human beings!

When Harlow is angry, she spins in circles and chases her busy tail. She just did that again and knocked her legs out beneath her, landing flat on her face. I know I shouldn't laugh, but that was hilarious.

I named her Harlow after Jean Harlow, who also had a rough start to life and died very young. My puppy was abused in her first home, taken away by an animal control agency, and placed in a shelter. Her previous owners were given the option of returning for her, but they did not. They chose to abandon her in the shelter, leaving her to be euthanized. She was one hour from death when the shelter called a German shepherd rescue service. Why were the owners even given a chance to reclaim her? I ask myself that question quite a bit. I believe she had been starved. She is still very thin, drinks rainwater, and eats insects. She has been freed of the many burrs found in her fur. Yet she is such a good-natured dog. How can animals that trust human beings so much, only to be wronged, be so resilient? I will never know.

Dan and I are working with the intake unit at his hospital to try a pilot program to foster animals that do not have proper care. I was supremely fortunate to have a dog-sitter who cared about the well-being of my pets while I was in inpatient therapy for so long. It is important to me, and those who are critically ill, that their pet(s) be well treated. The dean at my college lost a dog to dehydration because no one intervened while he was on vacation. That will not happen in my purview. My nagging fear is that a beloved pet will end up in a shelter, starved or dehydrated because its owner does not have resources to care for a pet during recovery. Quality care for a pet is an asset to recovery.

My plan is to have a rubric presented during the intake process at hospitals to discover if there are any pets in the home and if there is a plan for their care. Perhaps Harlow was destined to be my role model. I have already recruited people to help me in this endeavor. No one foresees critical illness, and it is important that animals are looked after.

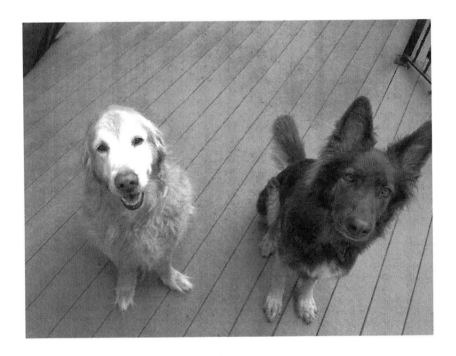

CHAPTER 12

Filters and Stressors

I have no filter now. Let's face it, I didn't have a very tactful one before, but now, it is nearly impossible to hold my tongue or avoid being brutally honest. I cannot explain why this occurs. People either love that or hate it, but no one has explained why I have no filter. If you're being an ass, I'll tell you. If I think you're lying, I'll tell you (and I've been so right when I am being fed a spoonful of BS. I was always a horrible liar, but I don't think I even have the ability to lie anymore, which is fine with me). If I've finished with any particular conversation, I'll tell you. When I have finished talking about something, I'm *through*. Forever. Deal with it, or don't.

Brain trauma patients have no room for anyone or anything that causes them stress. My situation is stressful enough, and I don't need anyone or anything standing in the way of my recovery. I realize that this phenomenon sounds like a petulant child, arms crossed, foot tapping, nose turned up. I assure you, it is not that. Many people in the early stages of recovery report the same thing. Anyone who knew me before will tell you I was relatively easy going and simple to get along with, but I am certainly more frustrated than before my illness.

It is true that I take out frustration and anger on people I care about the most. I try not to, but it becomes overwhelming at times. I think that is human nature, because the people who love me *should* be there no matter what. But oh boy, is that assumption wrong. I recently began to text someone who had angered me; I was enraged but in mid-text I suddenly realized I just didn't care enough. With a stroke, everything seems to go off and on like a light switch, so I hope this too shall pass.

The danger of depression is very real. I was never a depressed person before my trauma, so it is really troubling. I tried to remain optimistic for so long, but it is easy to become frustrated when reality sinks in. I still try to be as positive as I can under the circumstances, and I think I succeed (most of the time). I try my best not to burden anyone with my problems.

It is especially jarring and difficult to see pictures of myself before. I don't take meds, so I just joust with my negative feelings. There are times when I thought it would be easier to kill myself, but I am exceedingly curious about my torturous path to recovery and how this will end. Is it scary? Yes. Would I make it through another attack? Probably not. I will take it one day at a time (my new mantra) and assume there will be no relapse.

Numerous people have suggested that I see a counselor. I am a counselor! My counseling experience allows me to anticipate the techniques of a counselor I would consult. The strategies that would be utilized would undoubtedly cause me more stress. It also causes me a great deal of anxiety to rely on other people for rides, so I will not add the inconvenience to myself or anyone else. Added stress is not the intention of counseling. I do recommend counseling for people who think it would help them.

I don't like making plans in advance, because I never know how I'm going to feel on any given day. Pain is quite normal for me these days. At first, anything that physically touched me was painful. I have never been proficient at describing pain, but I would say that any contact would cause a topical pain, like pins and needles. Droplets of water in the shower and human touch were very uncomfortable. Fortunately, now, showering feels quite refreshing.

For a long time, I had a heightened sense of smell. That has recently diminished. For, a year, however, I was like a bloodhound. I could smell skunks and anything unusual from far distances. Even you, my reader, my have piqued my olfactory awareness.

I have fallen a few times, because a cerebellar stroke affects balance. My left leg aches much of the time. It is a debilitating pain. The first time I fell, I joked that I broke the fall with my face. I have injured my hip and shoulder. I broke a finger and a toe. I have cut myself on many occasions and have no idea how I did it. Such incidents have led to me to conclude I could be called a "hot mess." My best friend, Kerri, used that term once, and I had no idea what that meant. When people text me to check how I am doing, I usually respond now with, "I am a hot mess. Thanks!" I get it. My picture should be in the Wikipedia dictionary as an example now.

CHAPTER 13

Ugly and Dreams

I feel more unattractive today than before the aneurysms and stroke. Everyone has insecurities at times. I did before this ordeal, although looking back, I was in pretty good shape. Now I avoid getting my picture taken. I started grinding my teeth in my sleep and broke my front teeth. Thank goodness my friend is a dentist and fixed me up fast. I have nightmares about my teeth. I cannot do my hair and make-up the way I did before the trauma so that contributes to feeling unattractive. Trauma can make stroke victims ungainly and can undermine their self-image.

I have to wear glasses now because of my compromised vision, and I don't like the way they look. They aren't curative, either.

Sometimes when I am out I sense that people are staring at me like I am a freakish attraction. My response is to confront them, saying "I've had a stroke. Just deal".

I lost the ability to dream for quite some time after the trauma, but eventually my dreams returned. They are similar to what they were before the trauma occurred. I talk and write normally in my dreams. When I am dreaming I am never handicapped in any way. I talk in my sleep again, so that phenomenon has returned.

Generally, I go to bed a lot earlier than I used to and wake up very early. Sometimes I wake up at 2 or 3 a.m. and can't fall back asleep. For a time I staggered wraithlike around the house during these insomnia attacks, unable to see any better in the moonlight than the bright light of day. That phenomenon has gradually abated over time, and I usually sleep through the night.

CHAPTER 14

Coping

It is all right to grieve over the loss of the person you once were. From Ann Hood's novel *The Obituary Writer:* "grief is not neat and orderly, it does not follow any rules. Time does not heal it. Rather, time insists on passing, and as it does, grief changes but does not go away." This chapter includes coping strategies. I have incorporate many of them myself to cope with this stressful situation, and it is my opinion that these simple tasks can help sufferers get through traumatic times. Living in a rural area precludes me from having access to some of these coping mechanisms, such as a support group, but I would try anything to get better, faster.

o Talk to someone going through something similar or at least read about it. This contact probably was a greater help to me than anything. There is a wealth of knowledge in blogs, books, and research on the Internet.

It helped inspire me once I found that information. Amy, who is the author of mycerebellarstrokerecovery. com, was struck one year ahead of my incident, so it is helpful to hear what I can expect and what I have to look forward to. Many towns have support groups for stroke survivors.

o See a counselor if you think this would be helpful to you. Counseling could be helpful to anyone who has survived a trauma or for anyone close to the situation. Counselors can provide practical coping mechanisms, and they will listen with a nonjudgmental ear.

o Music can be helpful. Not only are some songs relatable, but also if speech is impacted, it is great for speeding up your rate and clarity. It is also useful to practice breathing. My vocal cords were also affected, so it is helpful to practice singing.

o Therapies. Such regimens can help with balance, walking, talking, and using limbs. The possibilities are endless, and a therapist can tailor a program to your specific needs.

o Keep moving. I have a lot less pain when I am not sedentary. Do whatever you are capable of, and you will feel much better. Amy swears by Kundalini yoga. Her instructor offers lessons on Skype if it is not available in your area. I am trying that now; I can't say anything personally about the positive effects, because I have just begun the process.

o Be as independent as possible. Count on those who handle tasks you are no longer capable of, but do whatever you can to maintain or gain independence. You will feel much better about your progress as you regain independence.

o Reduce stressors as much as possible. Stressors can impede progress, so as much as possible, reduce tension-causing situations or redact people from your life if they increase stress.

o Do what you love. I was struggling with feeling purposeful prior to my traumatic incident. I was involved with a local animal shelter, took cooking classes and photography classes, I became a certified ghost hunter and I was just getting involved with Big Brothers and Big Sisters. Most people who have suffered a trauma can't work for a while, or ever, so find what is fun or important to you and give yourself some direction and purpose. You will feel much more fulfilled, I assure you.

CHAPTER 15

Blessings

I figure I can view my situation in two separate ways. I can waste time feeling sorry for myself, or I can look at the bright side—I'm alive. I have solidified friendships with people I probably would not have met under different circumstances. I have learned, the hard way, which people do not matter or care. That is a good thing in the long run. I had a big heart, and I would drop everything to help a "friend" in need of help. I now know which of these people are truly my friends and worthy of my time and my heart has not shrunk.

I am thankful for those people who gave up so much to help in my time of need. I will be prepared to give back, someday, if I can. I am so grateful for the positive thoughts and prayers. I believe those help.

I think it is unhealthy to have a "woe-is-me" attitude for a long-term period. It's natural to be angry for a period. One is probably angry with God, loved ones, or someone. Let it go, eventually. Determination and a positive attitude will be catapults to overcoming any significant injury. People have been through worse things. It will get better.

I firmly believe we are only dealt what we can handle. I am certain that some people could not deal with these life-altering changes. There is a purpose for everything happening the way it does. If you survived, you were meant to survive. Perhaps just telling your story or relating to someone going through similar life events may be a lifesaver for some. That was a game-changer for me. I was a mess until I found a person to whom I could relate. She does not credit herself with saving my life, but I give her recognition for that. I was incredibly depressed and suicidal, but that has dissipated.

Thus I vacillate between the view from up and the view from down. Although I veer from one track to the other, rather like a blind woman at the wheel of a car, at least I can identify my swerves and know to steer toward a commodious center.

CHAPTER 16

Today

Today, I am much better than I was a year and a half ago. When I read that recovery stops at six months or a year, I find that conclusion very disheartening. Not true. Again, everyone is different, but I am living proof one can make great gains for years. Don't give up!

My last angiogram revealed that the aneurysms are gone, but the problems from the cerebellar stroke obviously still remain. The fear of a recurring brain trauma is always in the back of any stroke victim's mind. I am very reluctant to tell anyone if something feels "off" with my body, because I never want to go through this experience again.

The good news is that I hardly ever cut myself shaving anymore, I cook almost every night (there was no way I could have done that a year ago), and I have traveled every month since February. I now walk assisted by holding the arm of another person (my vision problems compromise my balance);

sometimes I get around at home without assistance of any kind. I joke frequently that I walk like a zombie from *The Walking Dead*. I lumber along, awkwardly; I do not swing my arms normally yet, and my stance is very wide in order to keep my balance. I cling to walls, doors, or anything that gives me support. I will walk at full speed again.

I recently deposited my cane in the garbage for good. I told my husband, "It's probably premature to get rid of it. I'll probably fall, but I will get back up." I am sick of the stares I get when using it.

A year and a half ago, I was like a wet noodle at the hospital. Anyone who sees me now, who had no knowledge of my brain injury, might conclude I was in a bad state. The truth is, I have made a great deal of progress since my stay at UVA.

I have great difficulty writing, but I just bought PenAgain, an adaptive pen. It looks like a claw, and there is a place for my index finger to rest. It gives the writer more control than a typical pen.

I still cannot drive a car, but that's next. I am starting small, with a golf cart, and I am perfecting the golf cart weave. It's a purple golf cart, and I call it "Purple Rain."

I would definitely be accused of driving drunk if I got pulled over by the golf cart police. I would fail any DUI test that measured coordination. In physical therapy, I often joked with my therapist about tandem walking. Tandem walking is carefully treading a straight line with my feet very close together, one in front of the other, as if I am on a tightrope. I still am terrible at it, but even tightrope artists need constant practice.

Often, I play cards with my husband. He has won twice since last June. Currently, I do not feel like I am living, merely surviving, but I feel that changing. I am taking more of an interest in traveling, socializing with other people, and looking "normal." Normalcy is nowhere near what it used to be. I am just happy to actively participate in life. I am even considering going to an engagement party in a few weeks, and I wouldn't have even thought about that a year ago. I have heard other people mention "re-entering life," and that's a great way to put it. I'm slowly, but surely, re-entering life.

Last year, I decorated my Christmas tree in August and sent out my gifts. At first, I didn't think I would be alive at Christmas. Next, I just wanted time to go faster, because I thought I might be fully recovered by the holidays. Now, I am talking about this upcoming Christmas; I recognize that I will not likely be totally recovered. I have already completed my wrapping and shopping, but I haven't sent out gifts yet.

I bought a recumbent bike for my bedroom. I have a TV there, so I can do those exercises while catching up on all the shows I missed. Ideally, it will help. I still don't see, talk, or hear well, but that will improve with time. What gives me considerable hope is looking at the handicapped plaque that dangles from the rearview mirror of our car. It says, "Temporary disability." Temporary. Anyone can deal with anything for a short time and come out stronger when it is over.

I am thankful for what I do have and what I have accomplished. My life is very different now, but I am trying to adjust. I observe people take so many things for granted, and believe me, I did too. I realize now it could always be worse.

If you fall, get up, dust yourself off, and keep going.

Made in the USA
Middletown, DE
03 November 2018